Elder Al's Elderlies Massage & Exercises

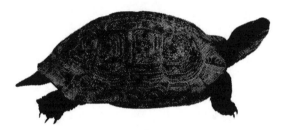

for 80 year's and up-

younger if you feel up to it.

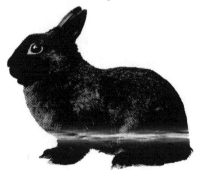

Order this book online at www.trafford.com
or email orders@trafford.com

Most Trafford titles are also available at major online book retailers.

Printed in the United States of America.

ISBN: 978-1-4669-1119-2 (sc)
ISBN: 978-1-4669-1120-8 (e)

Trafford rev. 01/17/2012

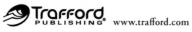 www.trafford.com

North America & international
toll-free: 1 888 232 4444 (USA & Canada)
phone: 250 383 6864 ♦ fax: 812 355 4082

Elder Al's Elderlies Massage & Exercises
80 years of age and up
Younger if you feel up to it

Before beginning any exercise program consult your personal physician about your bodies condition for your protection. Then if you decide this is the program...for "me". I want to do this exercise program. Do so at your rate of speed and with the exercises comfortable to you.

Remember proper breathing for you, for the exercise is important. I find it best to inhale when I start each exercise repetition, and exhale when I finish the repetition.

The exercises I perform daily, and have done so for many of my 80 years. Enjoy the exercises, and as you do-may the brilliance of creation, light life's pathways daily, with care and understanding...for you, in eternal and memorable ways.

Oh yes, I must also say, the repetitions of these exercises may be increased or decreased as your needs may demand. But do try to do the exercises. Just, to keep moving, what you still have– to move, its important.

Especially– if you're 80 years of age and up.

Now lets get started with the massage and exercise

The use of these massages and exercises and the
manner of their use is the responsibility of the reader.
The author shall not bear responsibility for any injury that
takes place while using these massages and exercises.

The Massage

At the start of each day, I find a quick massage a wakeful and a very relaxing thing to do.

It also gives one a chance to check over the body, bottoms of the feet, toenails, etc. After all-its nice to be nice, to your body.

My type of massage is performed, by you-by gripping, kneading with the fingers and thumbs.

I sit on the edge of my bed when I awake in the morning. You can sit in a chair, sofa, any place you find comfortable, to perform the massage.

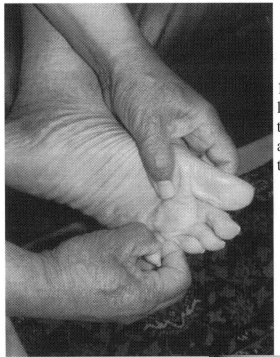

1) First I start with the left leg. Start at the base of each toe (I start with the little toe and work my way through the big toe).

2) Pinch along the base of each toe all the way to the tip. Pinch the toenail of each toe firmly (using the thumb and forefinger).

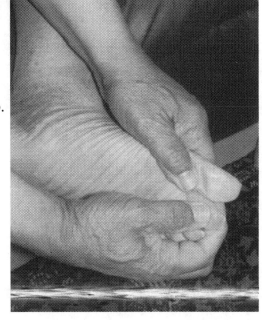

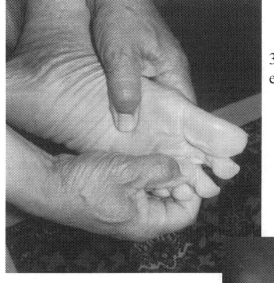

3a) Then pinch areas between each toe.

3b) Next massage bottom of the foot, starting with the heel grip the foot with your hand and massage with fingers and thumb

3c) Especially the thumb from the upper part of the heel nearest the ankle all the way across bottom, sides of the top, and all to the toes.
Go for it, wakes up the body.

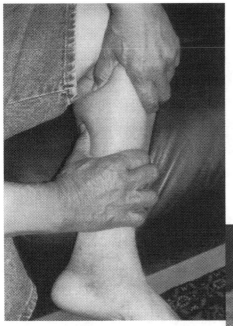

4) Next move up the leg from the foot, to the ankle, to the fleshy part of the leg to the knee. Massaging with both hands, thumbs and fingers to the knee (Repeat this same process with the right leg).

5a) Next massage the knee, gripping each leg with both hands and fingers, digging in good with fingers on each side of knee caps both legs at the same time.

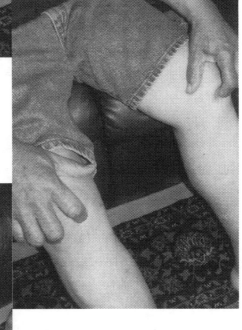

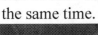

5b) Wake up those knees, thighs, cellulite, etc.

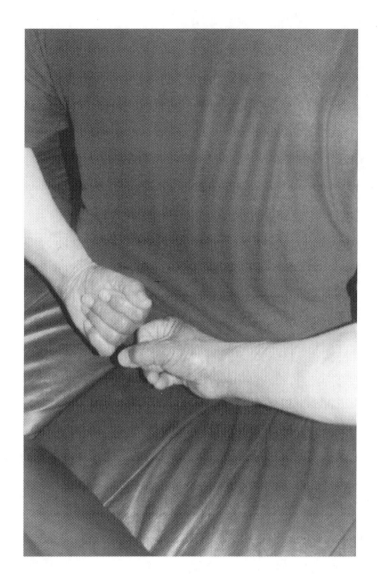

6) Next move around and rub base of spine, just to awaken it for the day.

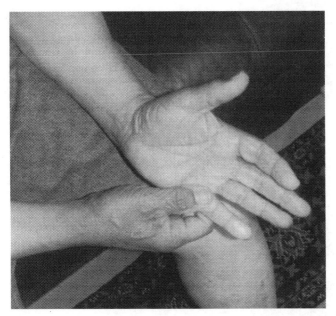

7a) Next move to the left hand massage each finger starting with the little finger from the base of the finger to the tip by pinching with the thumb and forefinger of the right hand.

7b) Pinch each fingernail firmly. Pinch between each finger firmly and with the thumb massage the hand palm area from the wrist to base of
fingers good. Back of the hand with fingers also.

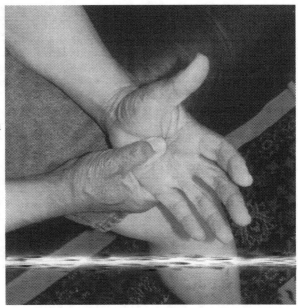

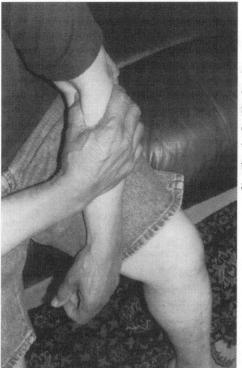

8a) Next massage from the hand all the way up the arm to the shoulder and where the shoulder connects to the neck. Massage with the right hand fingers and thumb by comfortably gripping and releasing hands.

8b) Repeat this same process with the right hand.

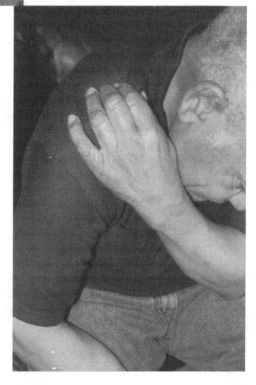

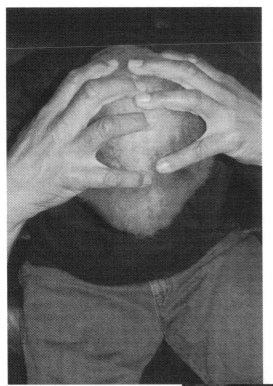

9a) Nest grip the top of the head with both hands and massage all over the skull area gripping and releasing lightly with finger tips.

9b) Also with fingertips from both hands, lightly massage neck area, grip release, grip release. Maybe for about 30 or 40 seconds or until you desire to stop. Then press fingertips of the left and right hands together 3 or 4 time. Finish by lightly rubbing your hands together.

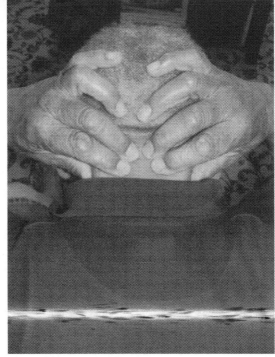

The massage is finished.
After doing this a few times to perform the entire
massage should take 5 or 6 minutes or as long as
each person desires.

The Exercises

Now on to the exercises.
Lets gets started with exercise 1 and move on from there.

Exercise #1

1a) From sitting position both feet straight down knees to the floor.

b) Lift and push left foot forward till the heel is even with toes of right foot and foot touching the floor.

c) Lift and move left foot back till toes of left foot is even with heel of right foot and foot touching the floor.

d) Do this for 6 repetitions. Do the same for right foot 6 repetitions.

e) Finish as in 1a.

2a) Lift left leg move it left from right leg about 12 inches.

b) Lift and bring it back by right leg touch floor each direction.

c) Do this for 6 repetitions

d) Do same with right leg, 6 repetitions

e) Finish as in 1a.

3a) Still in sitting position with both feet straight down knees to floor.

b) Extend left leg from knee straight out.

c) Bend leg at knee drop it lightly to floor.

d) Raise and lower leg 6 repetition

e) (on last repetition) Rotate only foot in circles Left 6 times, right 6 times

f) Then Lower leg gently to floor.

g) Do same for right leg.

h) Finish as in 3a

Exercise #2

At standing position looking forward

a) Spread feet to shoulder width
b) Raise hands to left as far as possible raising both hands to left as high as possible
c) Pivoting on balls of both feet, swinging waist, head, knees, freely till ball and heel of left foot is flat on the floor. Right foot ball and toes touching floor– heel raised about 2 inches.

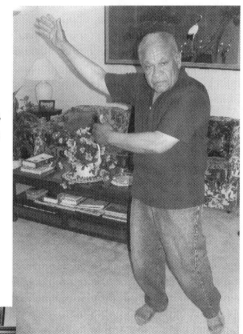

e) Then swing body to right raising both hands high to the right, swinging waist, head, knees freely
f) Pivoting on balls of both feet stopping pivot with heel of right foot touching floor and ball and toes of left foot with heel of left foot raised about 2 inches. Continue swinging left, right this Twister body exercise as a fluid body dance for:

50 swings to the left
50 swings to the right,
A total of 100
continuous left, right body swings

Exercise #3

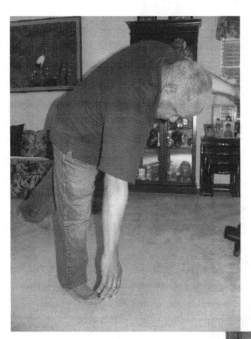

Step Back 2 1/2 to 3 feet and…
a) Lean on table with right arm- extend left arm straight out and down toward floor hanging loosely, and rotate arm in small to large circles from shoulder joint about 6 rotations clockwise and counter clockwise.

b) Then change arms lean with left arm on table and extend right arm, out down and floor hanging loosely and rotate clockwise and counter clockwise about 6 rotations.

Table, chair or other safe, stable, comfortable height support may be used in exercises

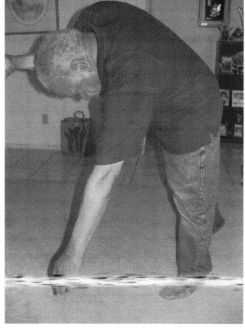

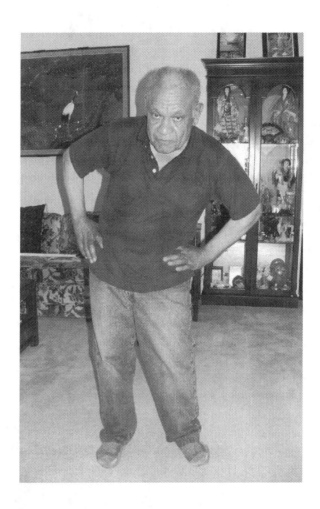

c) From standing position spread feed to shoulder width. Place hands on hips and from waist (keeping shoulders stationary) rotate hips from waist first left the right 6 repetitions each direction.

d) From standing position spread feet to shoulder width and rotate shoulders and hips 6 times clockwise and 6 times counter clockwise

Exercise #4

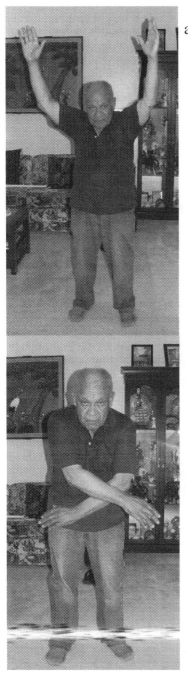

a) From standing position spread feet to shoulder width. Raise hands to shoulder height with open palms facing ears about 2 inches away from ears and push arms straight up. Then turn palms of both hands out, swinging arms out and down to their natural position each side of the body. Do this 6 repetitions.

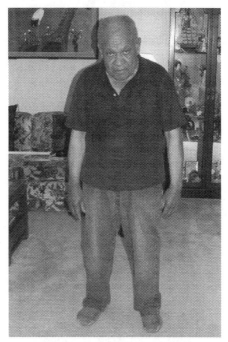

b) From standing position feet spread to shoulder width push arms to front of body and swing arms crossing arms over under left arm over right, right arm over left full swings 10 or more repetitions.

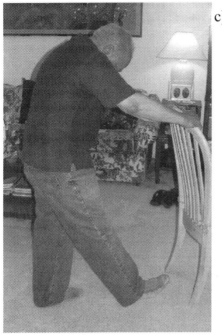

c) Spread feet shoulder width or more lean over table, place both hands on table for support, then step back about 2 1/2—3ft till comfortable for a good leg swing, Then swing left leg forward then backward about 8 repetitions on 4th forward swing stop leg and rotate foot at the ankle 3 times. Then continue swings to complete the 8 repetitions, with the left leg.

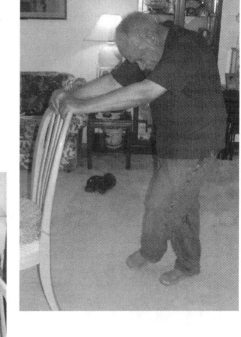

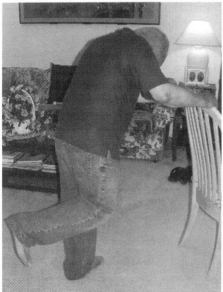

Remain same body position switch to right leg, do the same exercises listed in 3c.

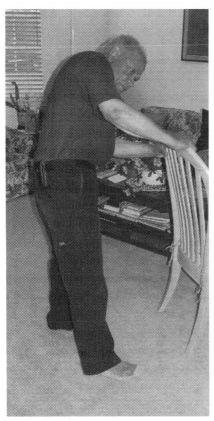

d) Remain same body position-Lean to right extend left leg, raise it to about 6 inches from the floor, rotate leg 4 repetitions clockwise from hip joint. Then swing left leg 4 times back and forth.

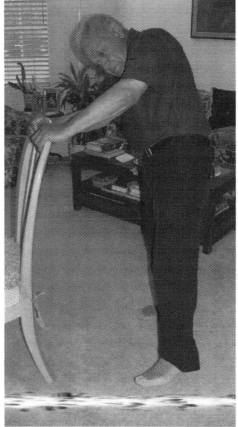

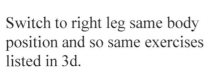

Switch to right leg same body position and so same exercises listed in 3d.

e) Spread feet shoulder width or more lean over table, place both hands on table for support move back about 3 feet or till

f) comfortable to do leaning table push-ups and deep knee bends. Do 10 table push-ups and 4 deep knee bends, bring knees down to about ankle height.

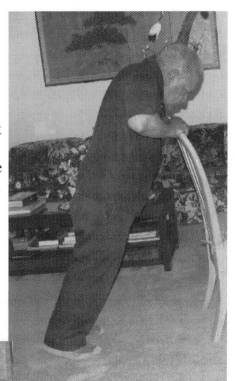

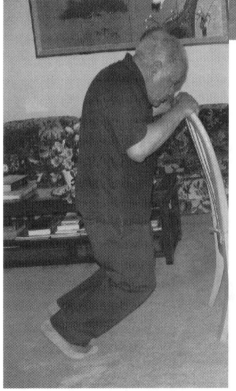

Exercise #5

Neck Twist
a) From Standing straight position– with head straight forward. Push chin down and at angle to left. Lift to straight ahead. Then push chin down and at an angle to right lift to straight ahead. Then "slowly" rotate head circular motion to left, then to right 3 times each direction.

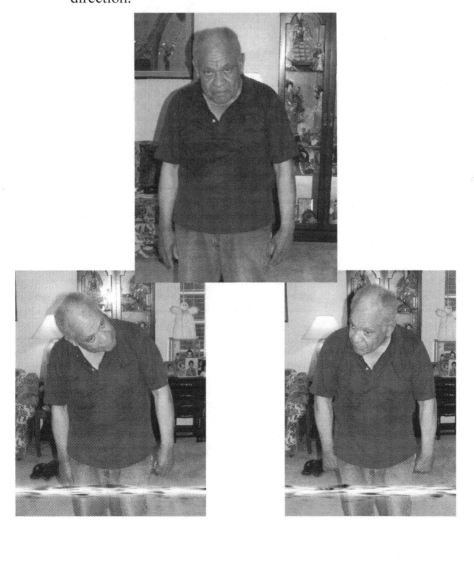

Exercise #6

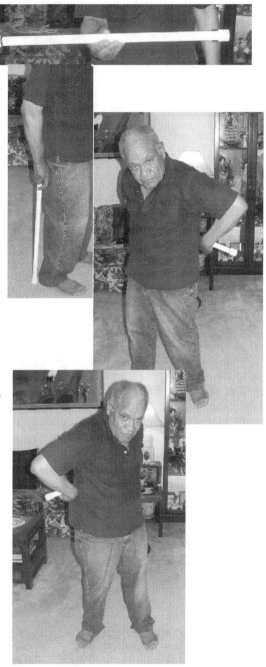

Bar Exercises
a) Make or have made, what I'll call a bar it's a piece of material– your shoulder width plus 8 inches for most of thee following exercises. Mine is made from a piece of 3/4 inches di-ameter lawn sprinkler water pipe with ends glued on it. They can be purchased at any Mon-terey hardware store. When bar measured length is decide, be sure it will permit the bar when presses on the floor beside your leg to permit arm to elbow to be slightly bent, to perform son of the exercises. Af-ter bar is completed-
b) Hold bar waist level in front of you spread feet shoulder width, and "holding bar" twist waist first left to right, then right to left 10 repeti-tions.

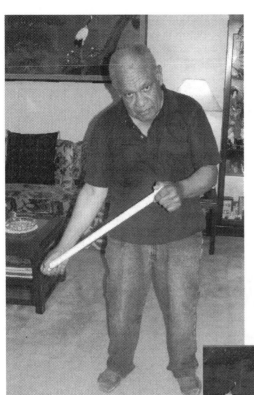

c) With feet spread shoulder width. Hold the bar at an angle across body, left arm at left shoulder-out, and extended up. Right arm should be down near right hip. Then… push right arm down, right arm up continue for 8 repetitions. I find pivoting on balls of my feet helpful.

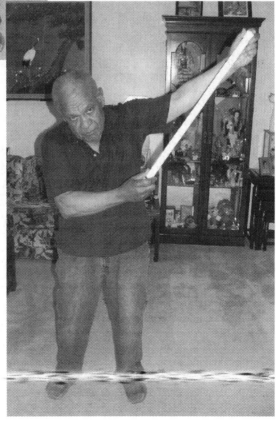

d) Switch bar to right hand. Push right hand up from right shoulder left hand near left hip Push left hand down, right hand up and continue for 8 repetitions.

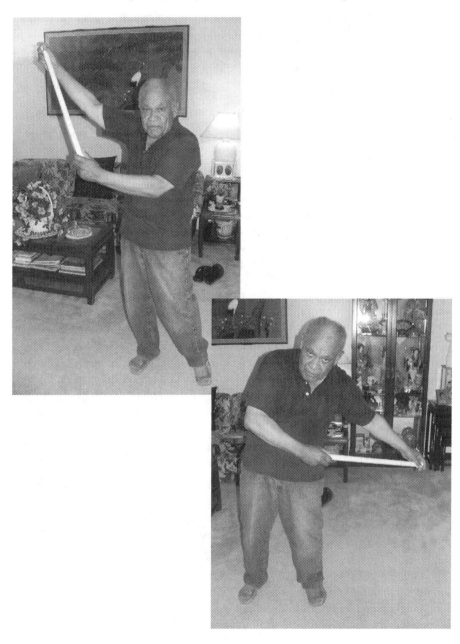

Exercise #7

a) Spread feet shoulder width, hold bar in left hand palm up, waist level in front of belt buckle. Right hand holding other end of bar in front of forehead. Swing bar down to right hip area. Raise bar back to forehead. Continue this for up down movement 8 repetitions.

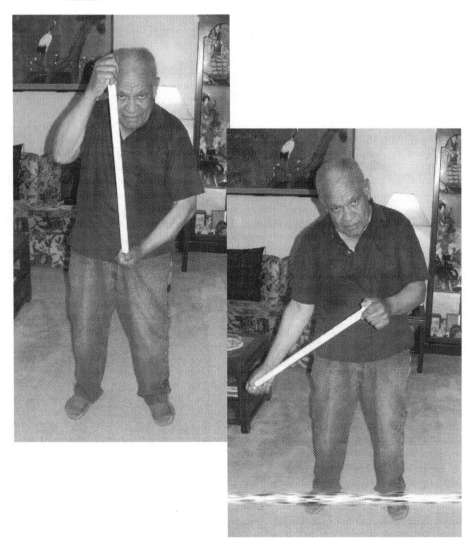

b) Then switch bar to right hand waist level palm up. Left hand top of bar near forehead swing left hand top of bar near forehead. Swing left hand down to left hip level. Raise arm back to forehead. Continue for 8 Rep

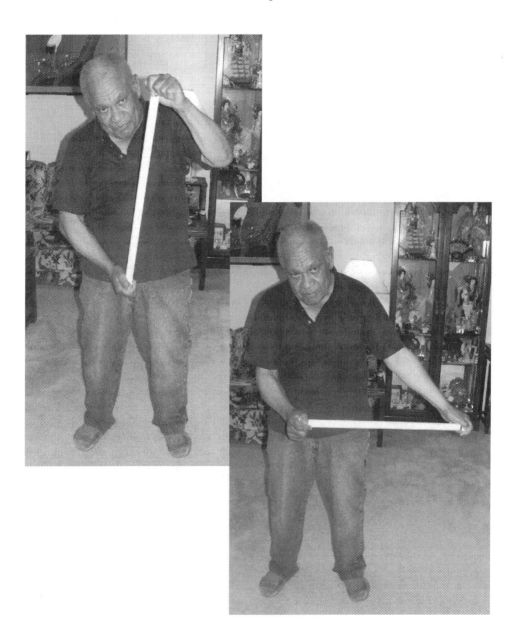

Exercise #8

a) Hold bar lower back, feet spread shoulder width. Twist
    Body left hand forward, then back and right hand forward
    then back.
    6 repetitions.

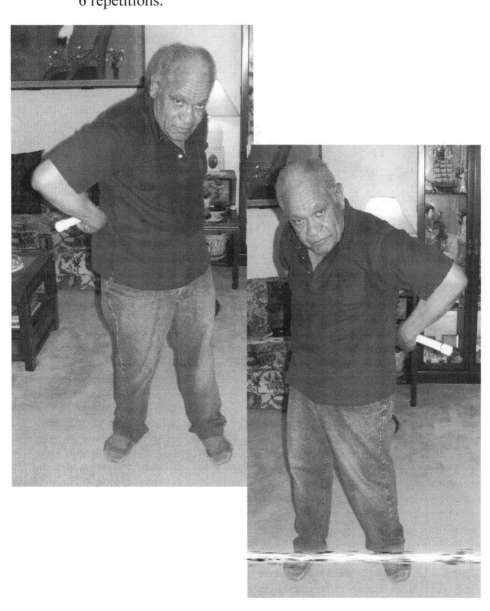

b) Move bar to upper shoulders, placing one hand either side of bar. Both feet spread shoulder width. Body standing upright and straight. Move left elbow down to belt level back to shoulder level. Move right elbow down to belt level back to shoulder level. 8 repetitions.

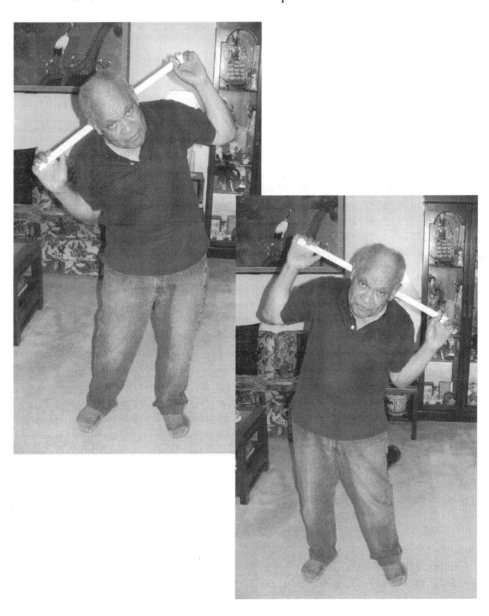

c) Then standing straight bar sill on shoulders swing left elbow forward– right elbow back right elbow forward—left elbow back.
8 repetitions.

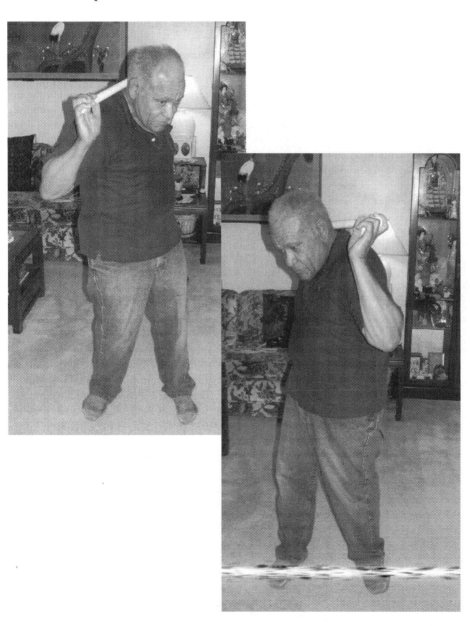

Exercise #9

a) Spread feet to shoulder width, hold bar in left hand palm up waist level in front of belt buckle. Right hand top of bar and squeeze– pressing bar top to bottom, flexing stomach, chest abs, and all upper waist. Turn bar horizontal continue to so the same. 4 repetitions each position.

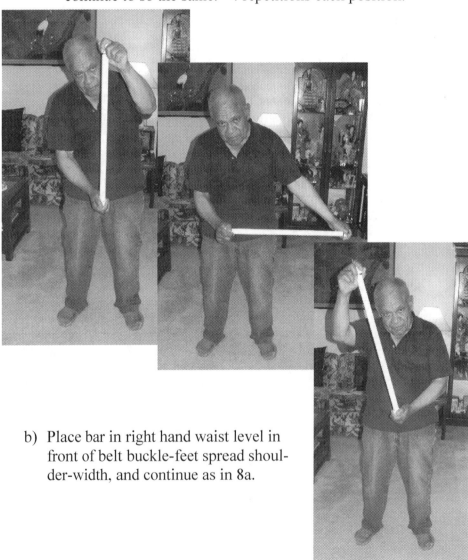

b) Place bar in right hand waist level in front of belt buckle-feet spread shoulder-width, and continue as in 8a.

Exercise #10

a) Standing feet spread shoulder width, hold bar left hand vertical position touching left leg and press bar on floor rear of left heel-flexing all upper body then move bar to front of foot to toe area do the same. 4 repetitions.

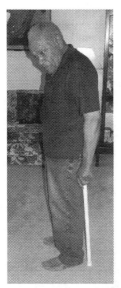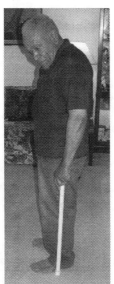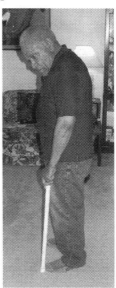

b) Move bar to right leg heel area all other positions as in 9a and to the same. 4 repetitions each position.

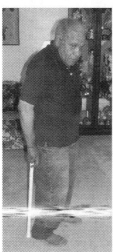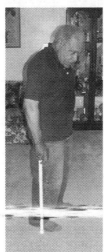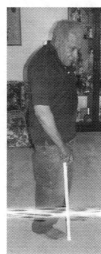

Exercise #11

a) Standing feet spread shoulder width place bar held vertically on floor, between left and right heels and press down on bar flexing upper body. 4 repetitions.

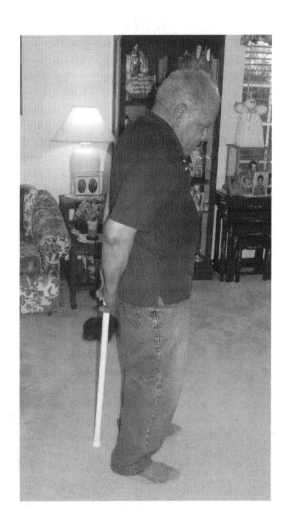

Exercise #12

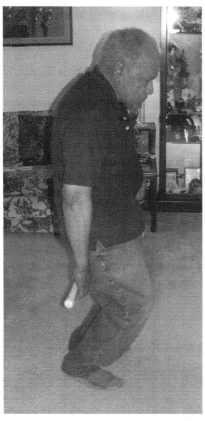

a) Standing, heels about 1½ to 2 inches apart feet at comfortable angle. Hold bar in rear, behind body– arms down palms out. Do 3 knee bends. Squatting a little lower each time.

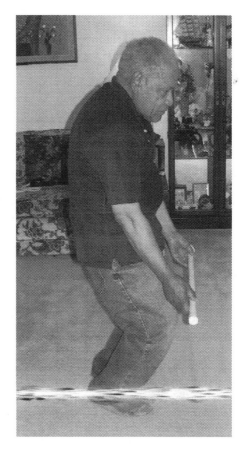

b) Standing as in 11a hold bar in front of body arms down palms in or out. Do 3 knee bends. Squatting a little lower each time.

Exercise #13

a) Standing feet together-arms holding bar in front. Keep body straight lean to rear on heels slightly and raise arms to front returning to standing position

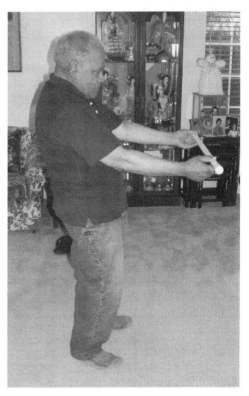

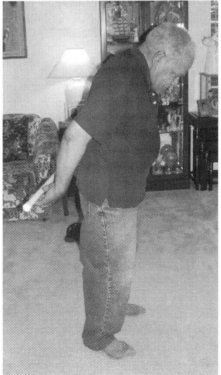

b) Standing feet together-arms holding bar in rear. Keep body straight-Lean to front on toes slightly-raise arms in rear to return to standing position.

Exercise #14

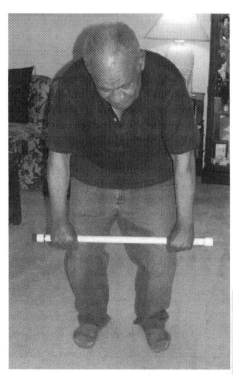

a) Lean over bending forward place bar between knees spreading knees about 10 or 12 inches. Grasp bar on outside of left knee-on outside of right knee. Then press with legs forcibly on bar against hand grasps.

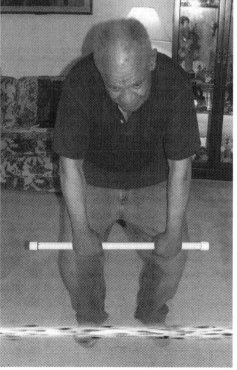

b) Same body position as in 13a only grasp bar hands about 10-12 inches apart on inside left knee, inside right knee positions on bar. Then forcibly squeeze against hand grasps.

Exercise #15

a) While holding bar in left hand with arms straight out stand on the left foot with right leg bent at knee and raised about 4 inch. above floor level. Balance on left foot arms extended 4 seconds. Repeat with right foot on floor. Switch bar to other hand and repeat entire exercise.

b) While holding bar in raised right hand left hand extended fully out from shoulder, balance on left foot 3 sec. Repeat same for right foot, left foot raised. Hold bar raised left hand right hand extended fully out from shoulder balance right foot 3 sec.

Exercise #16

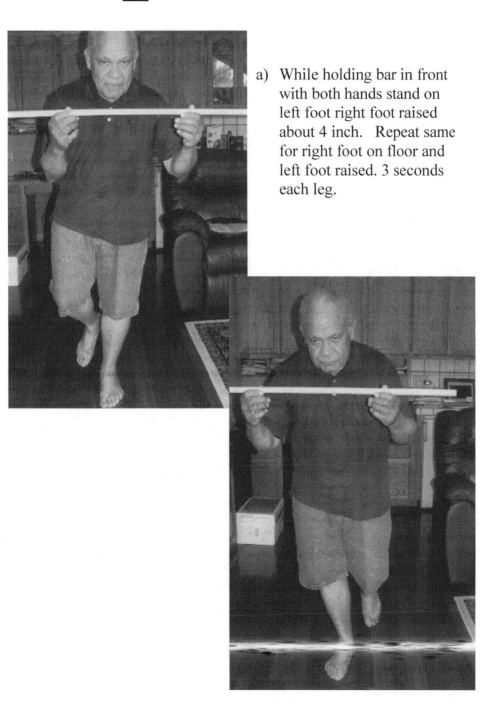

a) While holding bar in front with both hands stand on left foot right foot raised about 4 inch. Repeat same for right foot on floor and left foot raised. 3 seconds each leg.

Exercise #17

a) Standing with 3lb. Weights or lighter held at waist
   level raise weights to chest level 3 repetitions.

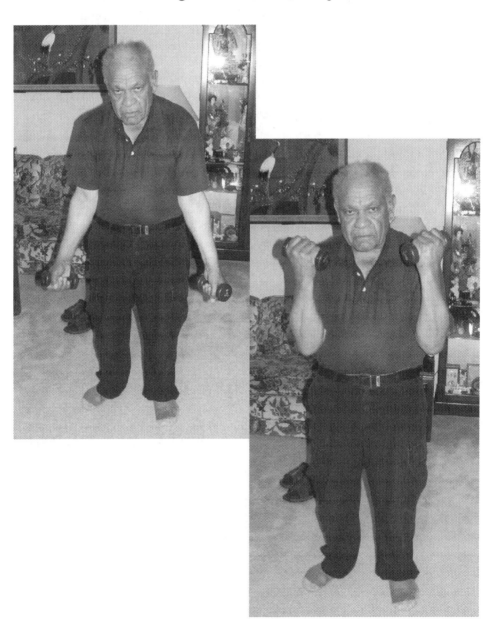

b) Standing hold weights at sides-raise weights to ears at shoulder level. 3 repetitions.

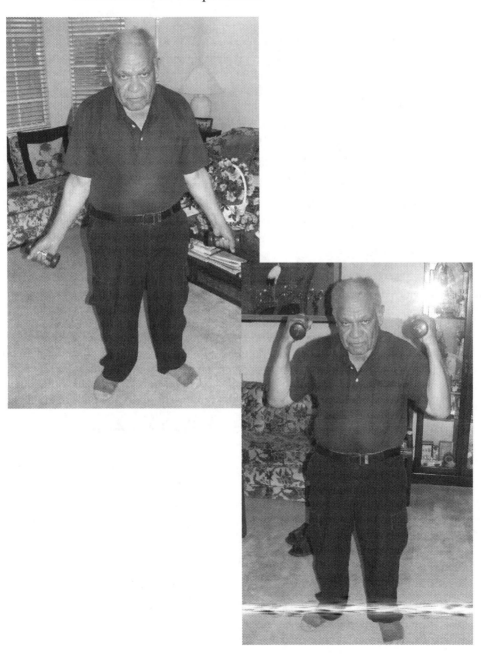

c) Kneeling– with right knee on chair left leg on floor–
   raise weight palm up to shoulder level. 3 repetitions.

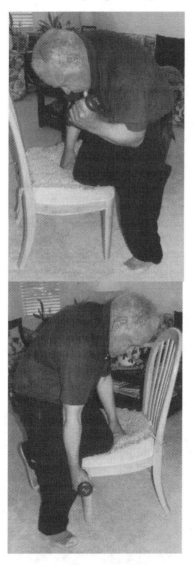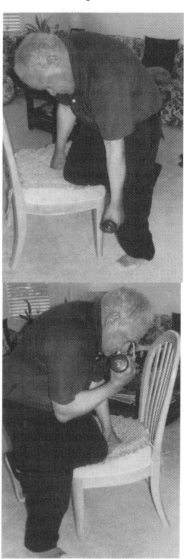

d) Kneeling– with left knee on chair– right leg on floor, with
   right hand palm up, raise weight to shoulder level. 3
   repetitions.

Exercise #18

a) With floor type hand grip waist roller.

For left hand   For right hand

Wheel

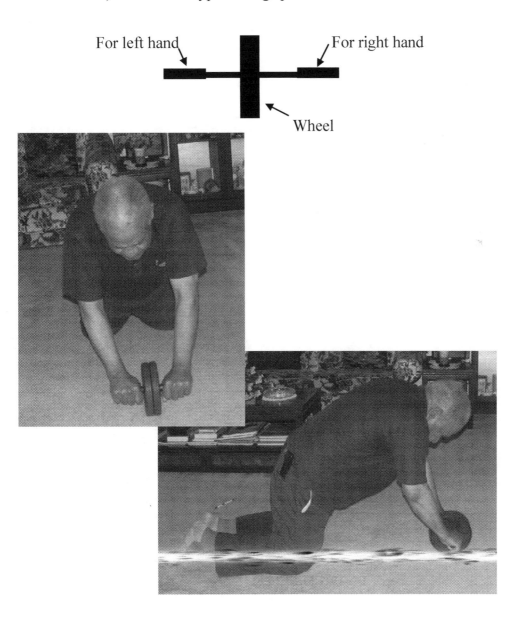

Kneel on floor and… with exercise wheel

Roll 3 time left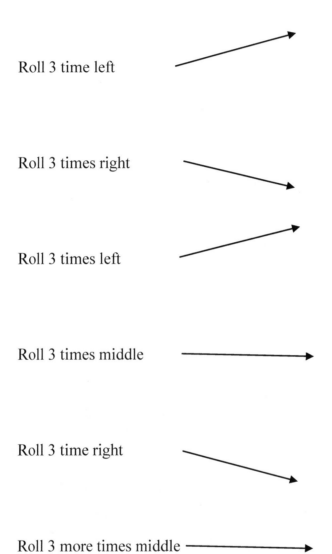

Roll 3 times right

Roll 3 times left

Roll 3 times middle

Roll 3 time right

Roll 3 more times middle

b) I find the small hand held exercise squeeze ball. Squeeze 8 times in each hand daily. Also the two roller exercise balls, held and rolled together with a flipping motion 8 times in each hand daily quite helpful   to improve hand grip, hand finger strength and flexibility. Find the rubber ball in most sport stores. The roller balls in most oriental stores

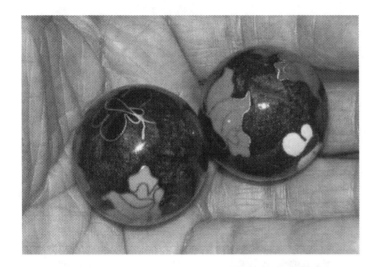

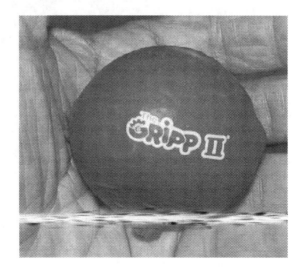

Exercise #19

With assistance of ab-roller, available at most outlets, perform 15 sit ups gradually increasing to 30.

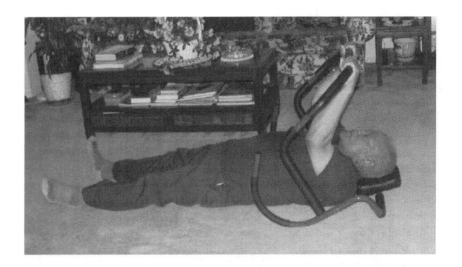

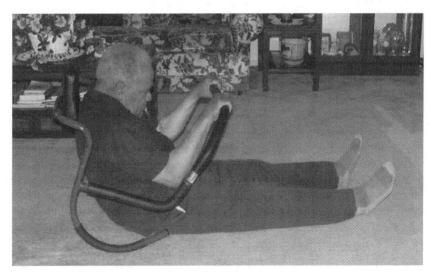

The following I do in the...
restful, quiet hours of the evening.

Exercise #20

a) Ride Stationary Bicycle– 10 minutes.
b) Regular bicycle weather permitting gives one outside
   air which is refreshing and great. "Enjoy, in legal
   place on highway" your speed, your time, anytime.

Exercise #21

Treadmill (your speed) 8-10 minutes.
"Outside walking is refreshing, beautiful, and good for
you." Enjoy your speed, your time, anytime.

Exercise #22

Skip rope (your style)
8 repetitions.

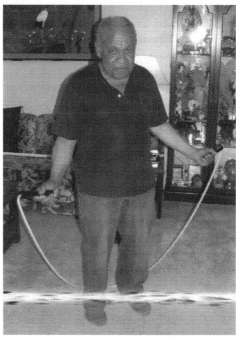

Exercise Notes

Exercise Notes

The main thing for all,
especially we senior citizens
is to keep moving at your
speed— what you have left to
keep moving, or it just won't
move anymore. Seems that's
a law, for and of, the ages.

Have a beautiful day, in a
most Lovely, Lovely Way

Al Vicent